IV STARTS
for the RN and EMT:

RAPID and EASY Guide to Mastering Venipuncture and Peripheral Intravenous Catheterization

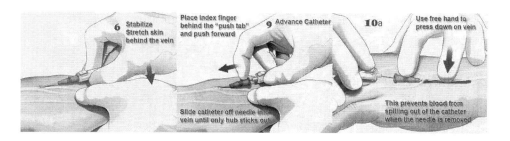

by

Team Rapid Response

Printed in the United States of America

Third Edition, 2016

ISBN: 1530479053
ISBN-13: 978-1530479054

CONTENTS

INTRODUCTION

Intravenous cannulation is one of the most difficult skills most RNs, LVNs and EMTs will learn. If you are scared out of your mind about starting IVs, you are not alone. It is an invasive and often painful procedure that requires both skill and practice to master.

Maybe you are worried about hurting your patient. Or perhaps you are afraid of appearing incompetent in front of the patient if you are unsuccessful. All too often it seems easier to just ask someone else.

Like any skill, some will be better than others. Some will learn faster, others it will take more time. **Our goal is to provide you a RAPID and EASY way to master the IV stick!** Not everyone will become an expert, and that's OK. But at a minimum, we want to impart every professional with the skill and confidence to start a routine, uncomplicated IV in their patient.

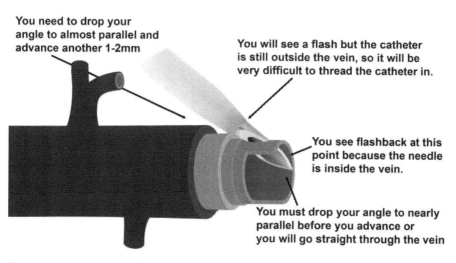

You need to drop your angle to almost parallel and advance another 1-2mm

You will see a flash but the catheter is still outside the vein, so it will be very difficult to thread the catheter in.

You see flashback at this point because the needle is inside the vein.

You must drop your angle to nearly parallel before you advance or you will go straight through the vein

Figure 1 – Example of Needle in Vein

This is not intended to be an exhausting comprehensive textbook on IV therapy; instead we present a clear, concise and straightforward approach to starting IVs.

We cover the following in this text:

- ✓ The parts and functions of different IV devices
- ✓ **Gauges**—choosing the correct gauge
- ✓ Basic anatomy and physiology of veins
- ✓ How to choose a vein and what qualities to look for
- ✓ **Strategies to distend veins** and make them **Pop Out!**
- ✓ Which veins to avoid
- ✓ **An illustrated step-by-step guide to starting an IV**
    - Specific techniques to stabilizing general veins, shallow veins, cephalic veins and hand veins
    - **Selecting the correct angle of insertion**
    - 3 approaches to insert the needle
    - The Y-bifurcation
    - **4 methods to threading the catheter**
- ✓ Guide to **the "Floating technique"**
- ✓ **Visual guide to what you are doing wrong** when a vein blows
- ✓ **Preventing veins from blowing**
- ✓ Finding and avoiding **valves**
- ✓ Inserting IVs in the elderly
- ✓ **Infiltration, Extravasation & Vesicant medications**
- ✓ Assortment of tips and tricks

By the end you will have not just the skills to start an IV, but the confidence to go out there and give each patient your *two* best shots.

We start with the basics for the novices who have never started an IV and for those who miss or blow most of the ones they try.

For the seasoned professionals we include advanced techniques and alternate methods.

We will guide you through the mess and help you get the stick so you can deliver the care your patient deserves.

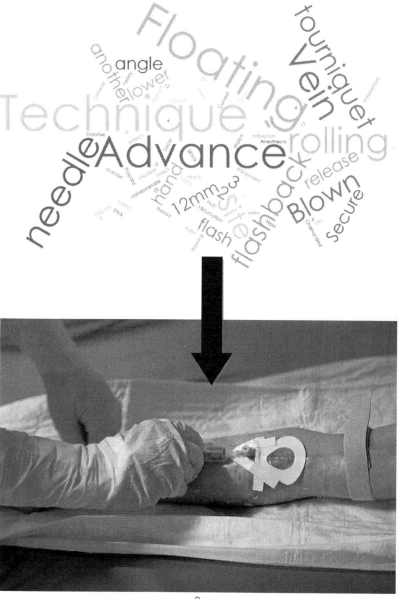

MEET YOUR IV DEVICE

There are two major groups of IV devices: the "Over-the-Needle" catheter and the Butterfly needle.

"Over-the-Needle" Catheter

The "over-the-needle" IV consists of a thin flexible plastic tube (*the catheter / cannula*) that slides over a hollow metal needle (*the stylet*). This is the most common device used to establish an intravenous line and can be left in place for up to 96 hours (4 days). They are manufactured with many different designs and safety features but the basic principle of a plastic tube over a needle defines the group. The terms 'catheter' and 'cannula' used to have different meanings but now both terms are interchangeable.

Looking closely you will notice about 1-2mm of the needle extends past the tip of the catheter. Remember that, we will explain why it is important later.

Placing an IV with an "over-the-needle" catheter involves four basic steps:

1. The stylet is used to puncture the skin and enter the vein.
2. The flexible catheter rides the stylet into the vein.
3. Once inside the vein, the catheter slides off the stylet and rests inside the vein.
4. The metal stylet is then retracted and discarded.

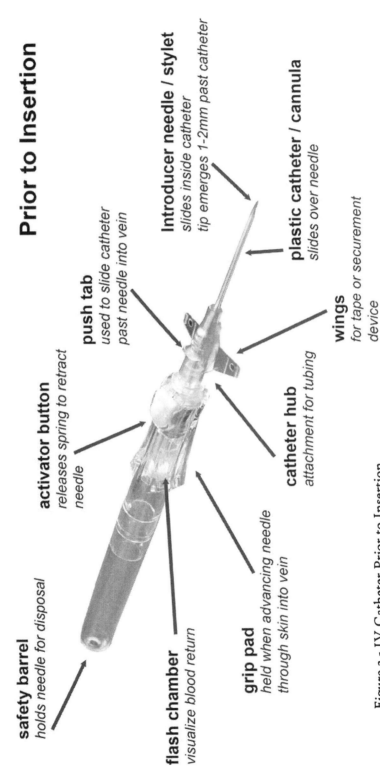

Prior to Insertion

safety barrel
holds needle for disposal

activator button
releases spring to retract needle

push tab
used to slide catheter past needle into vein

Introducer needle / stylet
slides inside catheter tip emerges 1-2mm past catheter

plastic catheter / cannula
slides over needle

wings
for tape or securement device

catheter hub
attachment for tubing

flash chamber
visualize blood return

grip pad
held when advancing needle through skin into vein

Figure 2 - IV Catheter Prior to Insertion

In the past, IV access was obtained by inserting a metal needle and leaving it in place. The limb then had to be immobilized. With the "Over-the-Needle" design, a metal needle is only used to gain access to the vein. Instead, it is the catheter that is left in place.

The risk of injury to the patient is greatly reduced because the catheter is a flexible piece of plastic. If it is inadvertently ripped out it will simply bend and slide out the same way it went in. It will not split the vein and tear a gash through the patient's skin the way that a metal needle would if ripped out.

The risk of infiltration is also reduced because the catheter will not scrape the walls of the vein when the patient moves their arm or hand.

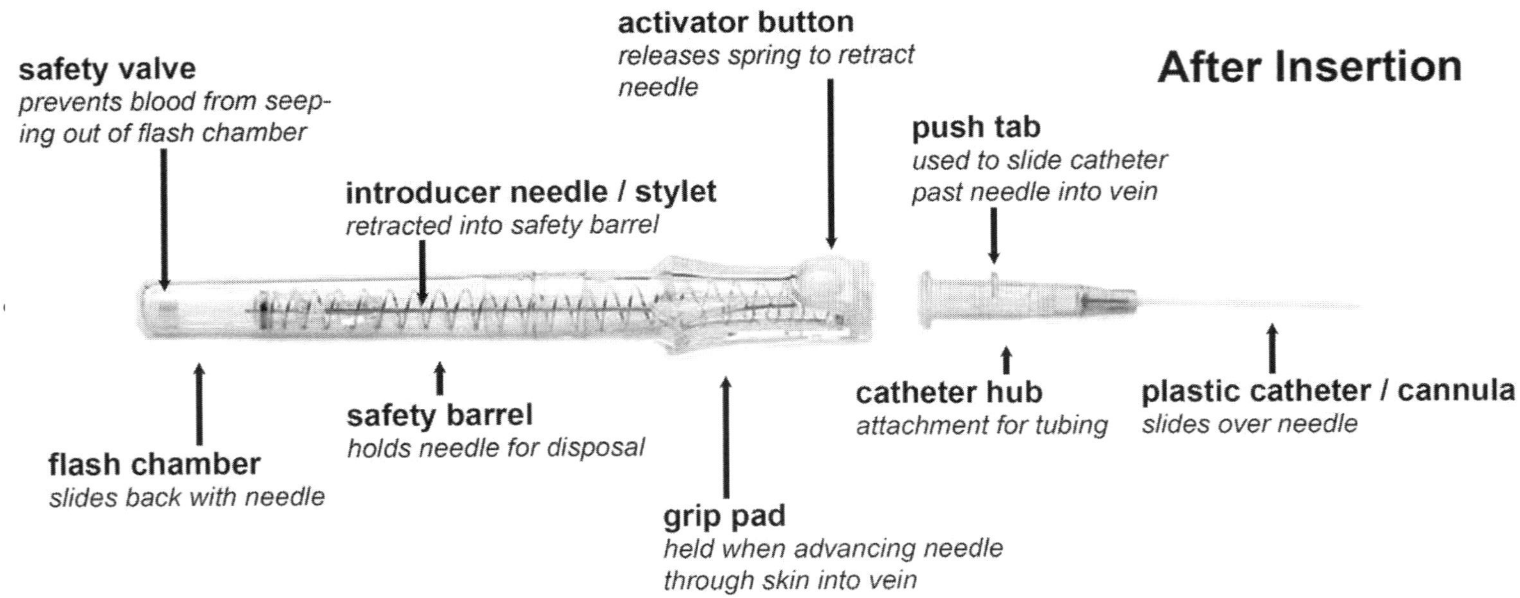

After Insertion

plastic catheter / cannula
slides over needle

push tab
used to slide catheter past needle into vein

catheter hub
attachment for tubing

activator button
releases spring to retract needle

introducer needle / stylet
retracted into safety barrel

grip pad
held when advancing needle through skin into vein

safety barrel
holds needle for disposal

safety valve
prevents blood from seeping out of flash chamber

flash chamber
slides back with needle

Figure 3 - IV Catheter after Activation

Parts of the Catheter

Catheter / cannula—a thin, hollow, flexible plastic tube that slides over the needle and is threaded into the patients vein

Catheter hub—provides a location for tubing to attach to the catheter. The catheter itself should be completely inside the vein, the hub is the portion that is secured on top of the patient's skin.

Introducer needle / stylet—a rigid hollow metal needle that punctures the skin and carries the catheter into the vein. The catheter slides off the needle into the vein and the needle is retracted back.

Flash chamber—compartment behind the needle that allows the user to visualize blood return, confirming the tip of needle is inside a vein

Porous Plug / Safety valve—semi porus valve located behind the flash chamber. When blood fills the flash chamber it displaces the air inside. This valve lets air out but prevents blood from spilling out when the chamber is full.

Activator button—safety feature on some IV catheters, it releases a spring that retracts the needle and flash chamber into the safety barrel.

Safety barrel / Needle Guard—holds the needle and flash chamber when activation button is depressed

Grip pads—provides surface for grip when inserting the IV device through the skin into the vein

Push tab—allows the user to easily slide the catheter off the needle into the vein with their index finger. Also indicates bevel position: bevel is up when push tab is up and clicks in place.

Wings—provides surface to tape down the catheter. Holes in the wings can be locked into special securement device. (The catheter in the first picture has wings with holes)

Safety tip—safety feature on some IV catheters. Rather than having the needle retract into a safety barrel, a specially designed cap slides over the tip of the needle and locks in place when the needle is retracted.

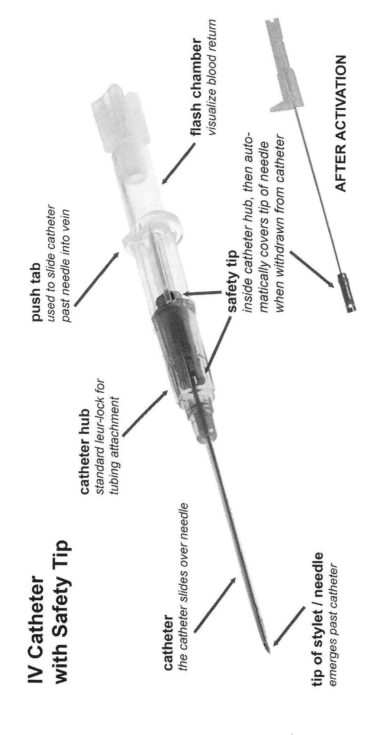

IV Catheter with Safety Tip

push tab
used to slide catheter past needle into vein

flash chamber
visualize blood return

AFTER ACTIVATION

catheter hub
standard leur-lock for tubing attachment

safety tip
inside catheter hub, then automatically covers tip of needle when withdrawn from catheter

catheter
the catheter slides over needle

tip of stylet / needle
emerges past catheter

Figure 4 - IV Catheter with Safety Tip

11

IV catheters are manufactured in many different styles and you will need to familiarize yourself with the one your facility uses. In particular, the safety features vary widely between models. The IV devices in the first two pictures utilize an activator button that releases a spring to retract the needle into a safety barrel. An older variation of this design does without the activator button and spring; instead the user manually slides the needle back into a safety barrel.

The third graphic depicts a completely different design that utilizes a safety tip. This design involves a safety tip that slides up to the tip of the needle as it is separated from the catheter. The safety tip locks in place when the user completely retracts the needle from the catheter.

Although the designs may differ, the purpose of these safety features are to prevent accidental needle sticks. However, no system is foolproof and it is important to always be cautious when inserting an IV. Remember to always wear gloves and follow standard precautions.

Tip!

The IV in the next picture has NO safety feature!

("Ported IV Catheter")

Ported IV Catheter

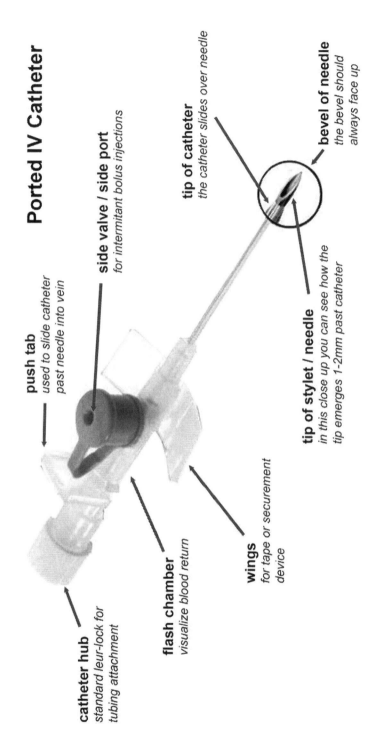

push tab
used to slide catheter past needle into vein

side valve / side port
for intermitant bolus injections

tip of catheter
the catheter slides over needle

bevel of needle
the bevel should always face up

tip of stylet / needle
in this close up you can see how the tip emerges 1-2mm past catheter

catheter hub
standard leur-lock for tubing attachment

flash chamber
visualize blood return

wings
for tape or securement device

Figure 5 - IV Catheter with Side Port

The Butterfly Needle

Also known as a "Winged Infusion Set" or "Scalp Vein Set", the butterfly needle is used for lab draws and short term infusions such as chemotherapy. Operating a butterfly needle is very simple: the user inserts the needle into the vein and leaves it in place. There is no separate catheter, just the needle itself.

This design allows butterfly needles to be made much smaller than "over-the-needle" catheters. They are also less painful and easier to insert. However, it cannot be left in place for more than a few hours and there is greater risk of injury if the extremity is not immobilized.

It consists of a small hollow needle at the front. The plastic tube that shields the needle is discarded prior to insertion. There is no plastic catheter; the needle itself will remain inside the patient. The two flexible wings that give the butterfly needle its name are used to grip the device when inserting and can be taped down to stabilize it in place. Behind the wings is the transparent tubing where the flash can be observed. The connector at the end can come in many different styles: a Luer lock to connect to syringes and IV tubing or a vacutainer connection for lab draws.

WINGED INFUSION SET

a.k.a
BUTTERFLY NEEDLE
SCALP VEIN SET

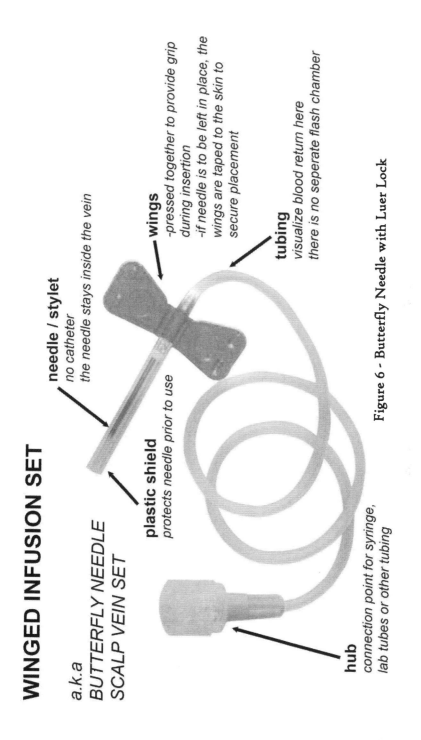

needle / stylet
no catheter
the needle stays inside the vein

plastic shield
protects needle prior to use

wings
-pressed together to provide grip during insertion
-if needle is to be left in place, the wings are taped to the skin to secure placement

tubing
visualize blood return here
there is no seperate flash chamber

hub
connection point for syringe, lab tubes or other tubing

Figure 6 - Butterfly Needle with Luer Lock

This design allows for more flexibility when accessing difficult veins because they can be inserted at a much lower angle and are smaller, thinner and easier to insert.

When used for IV infusions, these are more prone to infiltration because the sharp end of the needle can scrap against the wall of the vein rupturing it. Great care must be taken to immobilize the site and minimize movement as much as possible.

They are available in many different sizes, from 18 to 27 gauge. The 23G size is most common and used for lab draws. We will discuss gauges in the next section.

When performing a lab draw, if a syringe is used, it is important to slowly aspirate blood to prevent the sample from becoming hemolyzed. Hemolysis occurs when blood is aspirated with too much force through a small opening. The red blood cells burst open affecting the results of the lab test. You can avoid this by using a vacutainer to directly collect the sample.

Safety Features of Butterfly Needles

Many butterfly needles lack any safety feature and great care must be taken when handling them. The first graphic (Figure 6, prior page) depicts a butterfly needle without any safety feature.

Some butterfly needles do include a safety feature; this usually involves the user manually sliding a cover over the needle. Of the three butterfly needles depicted here, the last one (Figure 8) includes this safety feature. After use, the wings are pulled forward over the needle and cover it.

In the second graphic (Figure 7) you will notice a plastic sheath covering the front needle. Most butterfly needles include this plastic sheath to protect the needle prior to use. It should be discarded just before you insert the needle. Never place the plastic sheath back on the needle.

Some butterfly needles also include a rubber sheath at the backend. (The second and third graphics depict this, Figure 7 and Figure 8.) This design is used to connect the butterfly needle directly to a "Vacutainer" for a lab draw.

There is a needle inside the rubber sheath and when pressed into the top of a lab tube it will pierce through the rubber. The vacuum inside the "Vacutainer" will draw blood directly into the tube. The rubber sheath is a safety feature that provides some protection from an inadvertent stick when handling the device but it is not fool proof. If you were to press firmly against the tip you would get stuck! The last graphic also includes a plastic "transfer tube" surrounding the rubber sheath; this makes it even easier and safer to connect a "Vacutainer" lab tube to the device.

Of the three butterfly needles included here, the last one (Figure 8) includes the most safety features.

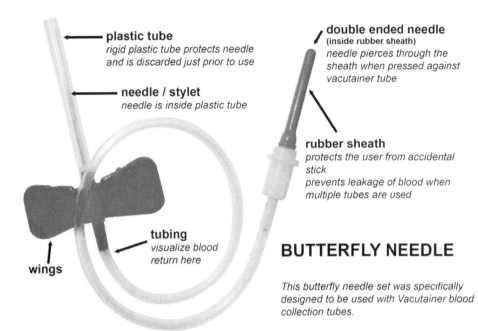

plastic tube
rigid plastic tube protects needle and is discarded just prior to use

needle / stylet
needle is inside plastic tube

double ended needle
(inside rubber sheath)
needle pierces through the sheath when pressed against vacutainer tube

rubber sheath
protects the user from accidental stick
prevents leakage of blood when multiple tubes are used

tubing
visualize blood return here

wings

BUTTERFLY NEEDLE

This butterfly needle set was specifically designed to be used with Vacutainer blood collection tubes.

Figure 7 - Butterfly Needle with Needleless Adapter

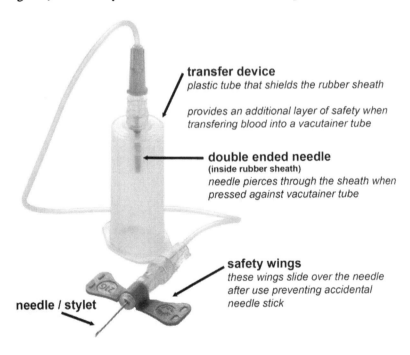

transfer device
plastic tube that shields the rubber sheath

provides an additional layer of safety when transfering blood into a vacutainer tube

double ended needle
(inside rubber sheath)
needle pierces through the sheath when pressed against vacutainer tube

safety wings
these wings slide over the needle after use preventing accidental needle stick

needle / stylet

Figure 8 - Butterfly Needle with Vacutainer transfer device

CHOOSE YOUR GAUGE

Choosing the correct gauge is the first step to starting an IV. You need to consider what orders and procedures your patient has now; as well as what they may need over the next few days. The size of the catheter impacts its function. Higher gauge needles are smaller and thus easier to insert, less painful and cause less trauma but they are also less versatile.

Gauge is thickness.

Needles are measured in two ways, *Length* and *Gauge*. Length refers to how long the needle is from the base to the tip. Gauge refers to the thickness of the lumen, or hollow part, of the needle. In other words gauge is a measurement of the needle's *internal* diameter. A capital "G" after the number is an abbreviation for gauge, e.g. 20G means 20 gauge.

It is counterintuitive—but important to remember—that **with needle gauges, a larger number is actually a smaller needle.** A higher gauge needle is smaller than a lower gauge needle. So a 24G needle will be much smaller and thinner than an 18G. Describe the gauge as "high" or "low" instead of "large" or "small" to avoid confusion. If someone says they want a "smaller gauge" it is difficult to interpret whether they mean "smaller needle size" or "smaller number gauge".

Lower gauge number = Larger needle

Higher gauge number = Smaller needle

Tip!

Don't confuse needle gauge with Foley or NG tube gauge!

As if it were not confusing enough, **Foley catheters and NG tubes are also measured by gauge, but they use a completely different system.**

Needle gauge is originally based on wire gauge. A low gauge wire is a thick wire. Foleys are based on *French Gauge*. With French gauge, a larger number means a *larger* tube. With needle gauge, a larger number is a *smaller* tube. Don't confuse the two.

What Gauge Do I Need?

The gauge of the catheter determines flow rate, i.e. how fast a liquid can flow through it.

With an IV pump even a small blue 22G catheter can infuse a thin liquid like Normal Saline (NS) at max rate (999mL/hr) so you could infuse a 1 Liter bag in an hour. However, you wouldn't be able to rapidly transfuse 1 Liter in 10min even with a pump; for that you would need at least a green 18G. If you are hanging a bag to gravity, catheter size will limit how fast the fluids will flow, even if you set it to 'wide open'.

Thicker substances such as blood products or albumin require lower gauges / larger catheter.

Routine Blood Transfusion?

Go with at least a 20G. Blood and blood products are thick and need a larger lumen to achieve an adequate flow rate. Imagine the difference between sucking water through a straw versus syrup. Additionally you risk hemolyzing RBCs if you attempt to infuse blood under pressure through a small 22G or 24G. To prevent hemolysis, you can forgo the pump and hang the blood to gravity. But remember blood can only hang for up to 4 hours. If it flows too slowly, it will spoil before it is finished infusing.

CT with IV Contrast ordered?

You'll need a 20G and it needs to be placed above the wrist in a large vein. The reason for this is that IV contrast is rapidly infused under massive pressure. In fact, the pressure can reach 300 psi; that is the same pressure as inflating a BP cuff to 15,000 mmHg! Or to put it another way, this is about 10 times the pressure in a car tire!

If this were attempted on anything smaller than a 20G the catheter could rupture inside the vein showering the circulatory system with broken fragments of the catheter. Or it could rupture the vein, leading to a massive infiltration. Neither would be good!

Usefulness vs. Practicality

Some clinicians advocate going for the largest sized catheter you think you can get. Larger catheters are more useful but they are also more difficult to insert, more painful for the patient and cause more irritation to the vein. Large catheters also require large veins. If the stick is unsuccessful and the vein blows you will not be able to place any catheter distal (below/upstream) to that site. Taking out a large vein will significantly reduce the number of available sites for a second or third attempt.

On the other hand, nervous and/or rookie nurses and EMTs will instinctively grab the smallest catheter available because they think they are more likely to be successful with it. This is also bad practice, you do not want to use a small catheter when a larger one is warranted.

Imagine finding yourself in the situation were you have spent 30 minutes and multiple sticks to place a 22G only to find out that the patient has orders for a CT with contrast and you now need a 20G.

Remember to always check your orders and think proactively what the patient will need.

Tip!

In general, a Pink 20G is a good all-purpose catheter and should be your default size for stable patients.

It is large enough to infuse blood products and IV contrast whilst small enough to cause minimal discomfort and irritation.

A small blue 22G is appropriate in certain situations:

- You are starting a second IV and you already have a 20G or larger
- The patient's veins are too small to accommodate a larger catheter
- There is no chance the patient will need a larger catheter, e.g. palliative care or hospice

When deciding on catheter size you will need to balance anticipating what may be needed against what is reasonable.

Sometimes what is needed is incompatible with what can be realistically achieved. If you are dealing with a patient with severe vasculopathy, give it your best shot but you may need to consider letting the physician know a central line will be needed.

Color and Function

The gauge of any particular IV can be easily identified by color. These colors are standardized and consistent across different brands and manufacturers.

See the picture (Figure 9 - Various Gauge Sizes) and chart on the next two pages for details.

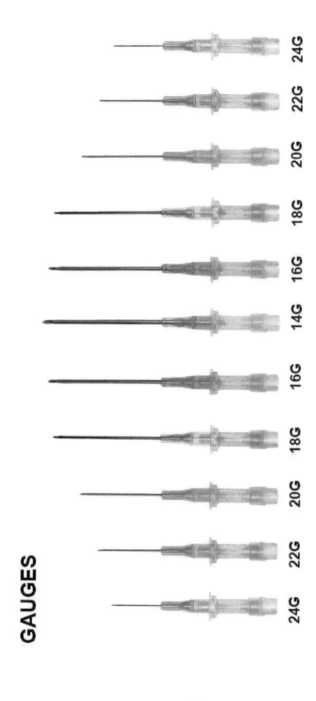

Figure 9 – Various Gauge Sizes

Gauge	Color	Function
14G 16G	ORANGE GRAY	■ High Risk Surgery ■ Massive Trauma ■ ER/EMS, OR, and ICU only ■ Largest size and allows most rapid fluid administration but requires large vein
18G	GREEN	■ Larger size ■ ER/EMS, OR, ICU, Trauma ■ Blood Transfusions ■ Rapid fluid infusion
20G	PINK	■ Standard Adult Size ■ Most common ■ "General Purpose Gauge" ■ Large enough for meds, hydration, routine surgeries ■ Non-emergent Blood Transfusions
22G	BLUE	■ Small Adult Size ■ Should not be used to transfuse blood ■ OK for infusion up to 1200mL/hr ■ Used for chemo infusions
24G	YELLOW	■ Pediatrics ■ Rarely used on adults
26G	PURPLE	■ Smallest IV catheter ■ NICU/Pediatrics

KNOW YOUR VEINS

Basic Anatomy of Veins

Veins are the blood vessels that carry blood back to the heart. Structurally, a vein is a thin hollow tube made of several layers of tissue.

Outer layer—*tunica adventitia*—thick layer of connective tissue

Middle layer—*tunica media*—thin layer of smooth muscle

Inner layer—*tunica intima*—thin layer of epithelial cells

Lumen—the hollow section in the middle where blood flows.

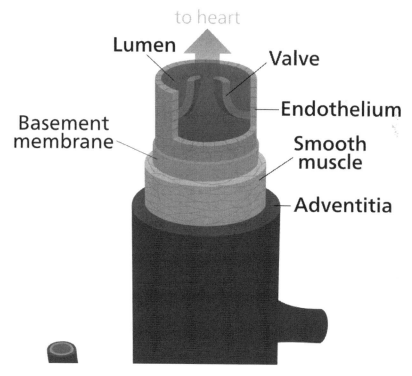

Figure 10 - "Vein" by Kelvinsong - Licensed under CC BY-SA 3.0

Tip!

Veins are usually not round as shown in pictures.

The wall of the vein is thin and floppy and will flatten out when not completely filled with blood.

This is why it is difficult to insert an IV into a dehydrated patient.

Veins of the Upper Extremities

IV sites on the upper extremities can be broken down into 5 major sites: Upper arm, AC, Forearm, Wrist and Hand.

The two major veins in the upper arms are the cephalic and basilic. These branch downward along the sides of the forearm. The **cephalic vein** runs toward the thumb and the **basilic vein** toward the pinky. These two veins are not completely separate and branch together in the forearm. The **median antecubital** (a.k.a. "The AC") lies in the inside bend of the elbow and is often a connection between the cephalic and basilic veins. The **dorsal venous network** lies on the back of the hand. It is interconnected and makes up the terminal branches of the cephalic and basilic veins.

Proximal

*Towards the body,
Away from the fingers*

Lateral

*Thumb side,
Palm forward*

Medial

*Pinky side,
Palm forward*

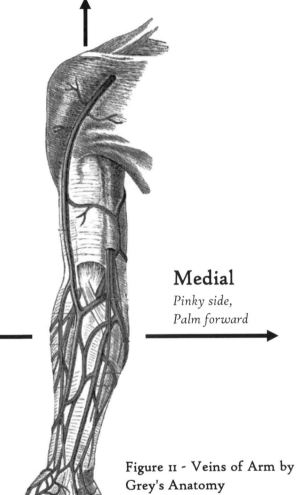

**Figure 11 - Veins of Arm by
Grey's Anatomy**

Distal

*Away from the body,
towards the fingers*

Tip!

Unlike arteries, veins show much more variation person to person.

These pictures provide a general idea but cannot be used as a map.

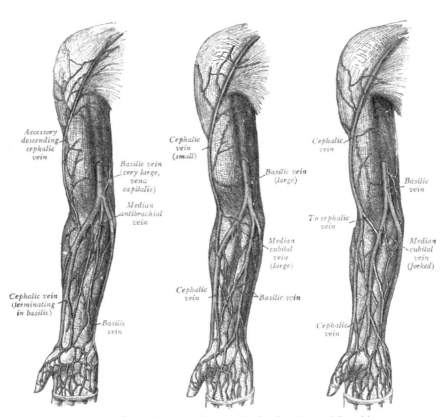

Fig. 597.—The most frequent variations in the veins of the forearm (schematic).

Figure 12 – Most frequent variations in veins of the forearm

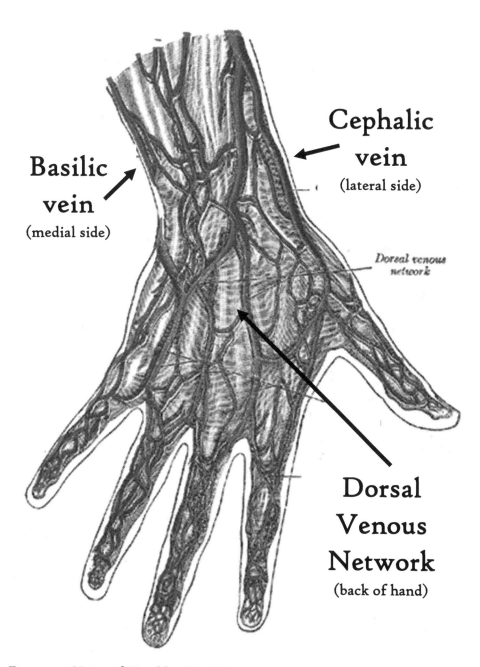

Cephalic vein
(lateral side)

Basilic vein
(medial side)

Dorsal venous network

Dorsal Venous Network
(back of hand)

Figure 13 - Veins of Hand by Grey's Anatomy

Other Sites

In general IVs are placed in the upper extremities. In some cases there are no accessible sites and an IV can be placed in a vein in the leg or the external jugular in the neck.

Placing an IV in the leg or foot is similar in practice to placing one on the upper extremities. However, these IVs are associated with a much greater risk for developing a DVT (Deep Vein Thrombosis).

Except in emergency situations, IVs should be avoided in the lower extremities. Placing an IV in the external jugular of the neck requires advanced technique and is associated with more risk.

MAKE THEM POP OUT!

There are many ways to make veins dilate enough to be palpated and cannulated. Usually only a tourniquet will be necessary; however, patients with difficult-to-find veins may require several approaches in combination.

Tighten the Tourniquet

Applying a tourniquet around the arm is the simplest method to engorge the veins. At rest, veins are mostly flat because only a little bit of blood is flowing through them. It is nearly impossible to catheterize a flat vein because the needle would puncture straight through.

When an individual exercises, their veins engorge to full capacity because much more blood is flowing through them. A tourniquet works by restricting the outflow of blood from the extremity. Blood continues to flow into the extremity because the arteries are not compressed by the tourniquet. Blood starts to build up behind the tourniquet filling up the vein and pressurizing it.

Start by applying it above the elbow to dilate all the veins in the forearm to assist in searching for a site. It can be moved around but should be at least 2-4 inches above the anticipated site (it would be difficult to thread the catheter under the tourniquet!).

The tourniquet needs to be applied tightly enough that the veins fully engorge but not so tight that arterial blood flow is blocked. Do not be afraid of hurting the patient when you tighten the tourniquet. If the tourniquet is too loose, the veins will not fully engorge. This not only makes it more difficult to find a good site but also decreases the likelihood of a successful stick.

If the vein is not fully engorged, the needle is far more likely to pass straight through the vein causing it to blow. Blowing a vein and having to make another attempt is going to be far more uncomfortable for the patient than a tight tourniquet and successful first shot. That said, you can make it more comfortable for the patient by applying the tourniquet over a piece of clothing. One method we like to use is applying it over the sleeve of their hospital gown.

Tighter is not always better.

Some patients with thin fragile veins are more likely to blow when the tourniquet is tightened too much. This happens because the tourniquet causes pressure to build up inside the vein. A healthy vein can handle the additional pressure but a very delicate vein may rupture the moment it is punctured.

You can often identify these veins by palpation. **Thin and fragile veins tend to collapse easily and feel 'mushy' when palpated** whereas healthy veins will feel thicker and spongy and have more 'bounce' or 'spring' when palpated.

Unlike healthy veins, delicate veins often dilate with the tourniquet minimally tightened. Try tightening the tourniquet just enough to engorge the vein but no more. Sometimes you may not even need to use a tourniquet.

Tip!

Never leave a patient with a tourniquet on. Not even for 'just a second' to grab another supply.

You can easily become distracted and by the time you return irreversible damage may have already occurred.

Blood Pressure Cuff

A blood pressure cuff can be used as an alternative. Compared to a tourniquet, it will be more comfortable for the patient. It will also provide more precise pressure control and spread that pressure over a larger surface area. This is beneficial to patients with skin that tears easily as well as those with highly edematous tissue.

Inflate the cuff to 40 to 60 mmHg. Sometimes you may need to inflate it to just above *diastolic* blood pressure or less, but never to *systolic* pressure or you will impede arterial circulation.

Use gravity to pool blood

Have the patient hang their arm down below the level of the heart. This forces the blood to flow against gravity which will cause it to pool in the veins.

Pumping

Have the patient open and close their hand making a fist to draw more blood into the arm. This causes vasodilation by exercise. Since the muscles in the forearm are forced to work, more blood is necessary to supply them with oxygen and nutrients.

Tapping and rubbing

Tapping the vein with your finger or rubbing it with an alcohol wipe will cause local vasodilation. Interestingly, the exact mechanism by which rubbing or tapping causes vasodilation is unclear. It may be related to release of chemical mediators (such as nitric oxide) from the wall of the vein.

Heat

Vasodilation can be induced with heat. Try placing a warm compress around the site and leaving it in place for a few minutes. If the patient has been exposed to a cold environment for an extended period of time, they will need to warm up prior to placing the IV. This can occur in someone picked up by EMS outside in cold weather or a patient returning from the cold OR.

This is a form of autoregulation that maintains homeostasis, called *thermoregulation*. Exposure to cold temperatures causes vasoconstriction in the skin, arms and legs. The body conserves heat by pulling blood away from the extremities and into the core to prevent hypothermia. The opposite occurs when exposed to hot environments. The body increases blood flow to the skin and extremities in order to get rid of extra heat.

Rub some Nitro Paste on it

Nitroglycerin directly induces vasodilation by relaxing the smooth muscle within the vein forcing it to expand. Rub a very small amount into the skin and let it sit for a few minutes. Research has shown a very small amount of nitroglycerin paste (smaller than a pea) rubbed on the skin will not have any significant systemic effect, even in a hypotensive patient.

SELECTING YOUR SITE

After placing the tourniquet, scan the arm for potential sites.

Smooth and straight, bounce and spring

The ideal vein for cannulation is relatively smooth and straight and will feel spongy or bouncy when palpated.

Bumps indicate valves which can blow if punctured by the needle or can block the tip of the catheter. Curved veins are more difficult because the tip of the needle may pierce through to the other side. Veins that collapse easily rather than bounce when palpated are fragile and more likely to blow or infiltrate. There are techniques to cannulating these types of difficult veins but the success rate is lower and they typically do not last as long.

Practice palpating veins on your own arm with and without a tourniquet on. Being able to discern veins from other tissue is a skill that takes hands-on practice. We can give you the basics in this text, but it is something that you have to get out there and do to become adept at.

With long smooth straight veins, you can insert the needle completely into the vein and then retract it leaving the catheter in place. This eliminates the need to thread the catheter past the needle into the vein. We will discuss this method later in the text.

Start low and work up

Think ahead. If the vein you are about to cannulate blows or infiltrates, you will not be able to use any site distal (below, or 'upstream') from the site of the injury. You would be able to make another attempt proximal (above, or 'downstream'). This is the reasoning behind "starting low and working up". It leaves room for additional attempts if a vein becomes damaged. So start by looking at the hand then wrist and lower forearm before going for the middle or upper forearm and the antecubital ('the AC').

If a vein blows, you may be tempted to start another IV distal, at a site below the injury. Don't! The vein may look good and you may be able to tread a catheter in and get blood return. The problem is when you infuse a fluid, the fluid will infiltrate out at the site of the injury above.

Superficial Veins

Superficial veins are near the surface of the skin and appear to pop out of the skin when dilated. These are easier to visualize and palpate but are also more likely to roll and move when inserting the IV. They also tend to be more fragile than deeper veins.

If you find a good superficial vein, roll the vein from side to side with your finger to get a sense of how much it can move. Veins that easily roll are more difficult to puncture. This is especially true if the vein feels hard or thick—the needle will push the vein to the side rather than puncture through it.

You can still cannulate a "rolly" vein but it will be more difficult and you will need to hold more traction to keep it in place. We will discuss holding traction and tips for rolly veins later in the text.

Deep Veins

Deep veins are more difficult to visualize and palpate but tend to be larger and are anchored in place with more connective tissue limiting movement or 'rolling'. Although finding these veins is more difficult, they tend to be easier to access since they are bigger and don't move.

Rely on your sense of touch rather than sight to find these veins. Palpate across the patients skin. The deep vein will feel like an area that has slightly more bounce or spring to it compared to the surrounding tissue. Then palpate up along the vein to get a better sense of its location and direction. Accessing these types of veins requires a deeper angle of insertion but you will need to be careful to level the catheter when you obtain flashback to prevent piercing through the other side of the vein.

Curved veins

Attempting to catheterize a curved vein is more difficult but possible. If the vein is not excessively curved, you can attempt to straighten it by holding traction to one side. You will need to be careful to puncture into the vein but not through the other side. Insert the needle just enough to get the tip of the catheter inside and then thread the catheter in the rest of the way.

Y-Bifurcation

Look for veins that bifurcate (looks like an upside-down Y). This is where two veins join into a single (usually larger) vein. The straight portion after the junction is more stable because the two feeder veins anchor it in place. This type of vein is less likely to roll than straight veins. Be sure to insert the IV *above* the junction and not through it if a valve is present. There will usually be a valve at the point where the two smaller veins meet. If no valve is present you can insert the IV directly into the junction. This approach will keep the vein especially stable and leads to less trauma on the vein.

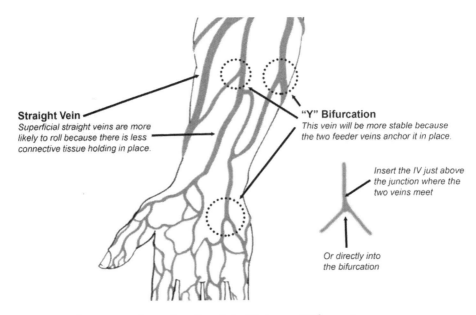

Figure 14 - Inserting through a Straight Vein vs. Bifurcation

SITES
TO AVOID

Veins to Avoid

Do not attempt to insert an IV (or check blood pressure!) in an arm that has any of the following:

- History of **Mastectomy** or **lymph node removal**—mastectomies usually involve removal of several lymph nodes. The remaining lymph nodes may become damaged if the IV were to get infected or by the meds/fluids running through it. This could result in permanent lymphedema in the affected extremity. Note that this is most common with mastectomies but also applies to any procedure where lymph nodes were removed. If no lymph nodes were removed then it is OK to use the arm even with a mastectomy.
- An **active dialysis fistula** or graft— the patient depends on that access for dialysis, damaging it is life threatening.
- **Blood clot / DVT**— the clot could become dislodged and end up in the brain, heart or lungs!

You also want to avoid inserting an IV through skin damaged by

- **Burns**—the site is more likely to become infected
- **Significant edema**—infiltration is difficult to detect
- **Infection / Cellulitis**—you risk introducing the bacteria into the bloodstream

Joints

In the upper extremities this would be the wrist and "the AC" (antecubital, or inside elbow).

Placing an IV in a joint increases the likelihood that it will kink or even dislodge. Think what happens when you bend a garden hose, the flow rate decreases or stops completely. If fluids are running through an IV pump it will beep and need to be reset every time the joint is flexed. If the fluids are running to gravity, the flow will simply stop.

A catheter placed in a joint can become permanently kinked if it is repeatedly bent back and forth or kept in a bent position for an extended period of time.

IVs placed by EMS and in the ER are often in the AC because it is generally the largest vein in the upper extremities and the easiest to quickly and reliably access. The AC can also sustain a larger catheter which is important should the patient need emergency fluid or blood resuscitation. A stable patient on the floor would be better off with an IV in the hand or forearm.

Blown vein

A blown vein will present as a bruise centered over the vein, you may even be able to visualize the puncture from the previous attempt. Sometimes they are easy to identify, such as a bandage over a vein with a bruise underneath.

A blown vein indicates that the wall of the vein has ruptured and blood spilt out into the surrounding tissue. If another IV is started *distal* to (below/upstream) the site of the rupture then any fluids or medication that is infused will *infiltrate* (leak out).

You cannot attempt another stick on *the same vein* distal to (below) the injury but you can attempt another stick proximal to (above) the site, or anywhere on a *different vein*.

Veins blow for many reasons and there are techniques to prevent this which we will discuss this more in the chapter: *Veins that Blow*.

It is important to be able to identify a previously blown vein before you attempt to start an IV because it will determine where you can and cannot start.

This applies anytime the vein is punctured, even if it does not "blow". For example, a working catheter expires after 96hours and needs to be replaced. Generally, the vein will not blow when it is removed but if the replacement IV will be placed in the same vein, it should be started proximal to (above) the old site or on a separate unconnected vein.

For this reason it is always good practice to start at the most distal section of the vein (closest to the hand) because that leaves the rest of the vein available for additional attempts.

Tip!

You can attempt to access a curved vein by stretching it such that it straightens out while the catheter is threaded in.

Twisting / Torturous veins

These veins are tempting because they often bulge out and are easy to visualize and palpate. Unfortunately it will be difficult to impossible to thread the catheter in. The walls on these veins are also weakened making them more likely to blow.

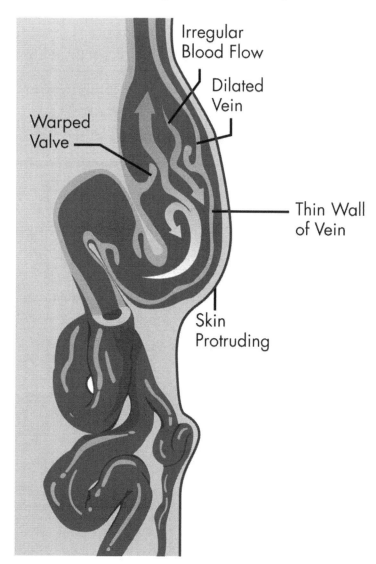

Figure 15 - Torturous Bulging Vein

Valves

Avoid inserting an IV through, or just below, a valve—it will be difficult to thread or get blood return.

They are often found at junctions were two veins join together. Valves appear as raised bumps along the length of the vein. If you carefully palpate the vein, you should be able to feel the subtle difference between the smooth length of the vein and the bump of the valve.

For more information see the chapter: *Valves*.

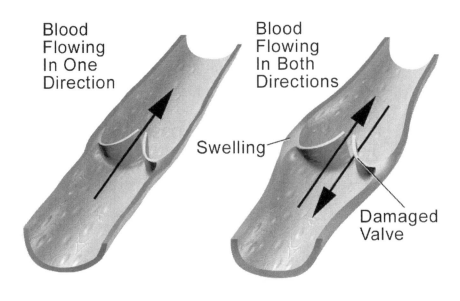

Blood Flowing In One Direction

Blood Flowing In Both Directions

Swelling

Damaged Valve

Normal Vein   **Varicose Vein**

EQUIPMENT

Before you attempt the IV stick gather and prepare all your equipment. Many facilities stock IV Start Kits that contain most of what you need.

Basic Equipment

- Catheter (bring a few and different gauge sizes)
- Tourniquet
- Connection tubing
- Flushes (at least 2)
- Alcohol and/or CHG wipes
- Sterile Gauze
- Transparent Dressing
- Tape
- Chux or towel to keep area clean

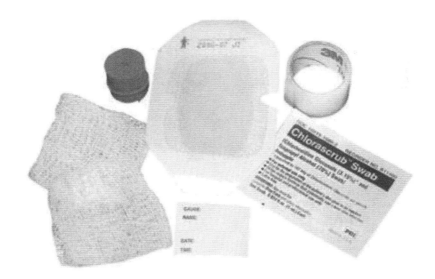

Figure 16 - Standard IV Kit

IV Start Toolbox

An IV start tool box such as the one in the picture below includes everything you would need. Organizing IV supplies in such a manner reduces the need to leave the patient to fetch additional supplies. This improves time efficiency as well as patient satisfaction by reducing the time spent obtaining IV access, particularly with difficult siticks.

If your facility does not have an IV Start Toolbox, create one! The one in this picture was created as a part of an evidence-based practice project for my unit.

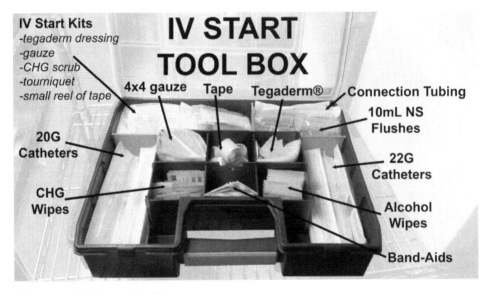

Figure 17- IV Start Toolbox

THE STANDARD TECHNIQUE STEP-BY-STEP

These are the basic steps to starting a standard IV. Each section will be discussed in depth and includes graphics and illustrations to help you visualize the process.

1. Prepare your equipment.
2. Apply the tourniquet. Select a Site.
3. Visualize and Palpate the Vein.
4. Sterilize the Site.
5. Local Anesthesia.
6. Stabilize.
7. Insert the needle.
8. Watch for the Flash. Lower your angle and advance another 1-2mm. Release the Tourniquet.
9. Thread the catheter
10. Retract the Needle.
11. Secure the Hub. Attach tubing.
12. Verify the Stick is good.
13. Secure the Site.

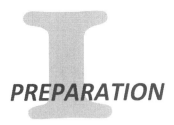

PREPARATION

First introduce yourself to the patient and explain that you are going to start an IV. Do not say, "I'm going to *try* to start an IV." That implies self-doubt and a lack of self-confidence. The patient will be more comfortable if you look and sound like you know what you are doing.

Prepare your equipment:

- Open up all the packaging and make sure everything is within reach.
- Prepare a small strip of tape to secure the catheter.
- Attach a flush to the connection tubing and/or hub and prime it. You may also want to loosen the cap on the tubing so that you can later remove it with just one hand.
- Place Chux or towel under the patients arm. This serves two purposes: it provides a clean surface to place equipment on and will catch any blood that would otherwise spill on the patient or bed/stretcher.
- Sometimes it can be helpful to place a pillow under the patient's arm. This will raise their arm up and allow you to visualize the veins and insert the IV more easily.

2 APPLY THE TOURNIQUET
SELECT A SITE

Apply the tourniquet above the elbow and scan the arm for a good vein.

If you cannot find any good veins use the techniques discussed earlier to induce vasodilation and engorge the veins.

- Drop the arm below the level of the heart and let gravity pool blood in the veins
- Have them open and close their hand rapidly
- Rub the arm or vein with an alcohol or CHG wipe
- Apply a warm compress
- Try using a blood pressure cuff
- Rub a tiny amount of nitroglycerin ointment over the vein
- Move the tourniquet to another site.

Above the wrist, below the elbow, above the elbow. Try the other arm.

Remember, you want to start low and work your way up. So start looking at the hand, wrist then lower forearm and upper forearm. This is especially important if the patient looks like they are going to be a difficult stick and you (and/or others) will need to make multiple attempts. If you blow a vein in the forearm, you will not be able to use any vein in the hand that feeds into the blown vein. But if a vein in the hand blows, you will still be able to use the same vein above the site of injury.

If a vein blows, you can always attempt another stick on the same vein above / proximal to the previous stick but never below. Remember to hold pressure on the vein for a few minutes if it blows to prevent a large bruise from forming.

Review the chapters: *Selecting a Site* and *Make them Pop Out!*

3

VISUALIZE AND PALPATE THE VEIN

Palpate up the length of the vein to get a feel for it. The ideal vein will be relatively straight and smooth, and you want to feel a slight spring or bounce when pressed.

You can use the needle to approximate how far the catheter will sit inside the vein.

Avoid valves and torturous veins. Valves will feel and/or look like bumps along the length of the vein. You can place the IV just above the bump as long as there is enough room between valves for the catheter.

Surface veins are easy to visualize but more likely to roll. Use your finger to push the vein side-to-side to get a feel for how much it moves. You will need to apply counter-traction to these types of veins.

Deep veins are difficult to visualize but larger and more stable. To find these, palpate across the skin, feeling for an area that has more 'bounce' or 'spring' than the surrounding skin. Depending how deep the vein is, you may be able to visualize them as a slight rise in the skin that extends in a line up the length of the arm.

Oftentimes it is easier to visualize the vein after sterilizing it with an alcohol wipe. The scrubbing/rubbing action causes some direct vasodilation. Additionally, getting the skin wet with alcohol makes the vein appear more prominent.

Tip!

Trust your fingers over your eyes.

You will have better luck cannulating a vein that you cannot see but feels round and bouncy.

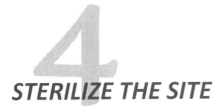

STERILIZE THE SITE

Now that you have zeroed in on your site you need to sterilize it.

Scrub the selected site with a Chlorhexidine (CHG) or an alcohol wipe for 30-60 seconds. Then allow it to dry. The bacteria on the patient's skin do not instantly die when exposed to alcohol. It takes several seconds, so that is why it is important to let the alcohol/CHG dry. The other reason is that if you insert the needle while the skin is still wet with alcohol, some of the alcohol will be drawn in with the needle and will cause additional stinging and burning.

If you touch the site after cleaning, you will have to clean it again.

Avoid the compulsion to touch the site "one last time" just before inserting the needle. If you find yourself doing this, it is probably because you are not sure of the location of the vein. Instead, mark the site by pressing your fingernail into the skin directly over the vein. You will need sterilize the site again but your fingernail should leave an impression to guide inserting the IV in the correct location.

CHG vs. Alcohol

Opt for chlorhexidine gluconate (CHG) over a simple alcohol wipe if you have the choice. CHG wipes have 70% alcohol just like a standard alcohol wipe but they are also infused with 2% chlorhexidine gluconate. This leaves a film on the skin that will continue to kill microbes for about 48 hours.

This is important because an alcohol wipe can never kill all the bacteria on the skin. Some survive and start multiplying the moment the alcohol dries. The film that the CHG wipe leaves behind will continue killing bacteria for another two days. This further reduces the chance of an infection colonizing the catheter site and the resulting bacterial phlebitis.

Scrub, scrub, scrub

You will need to really scrub the site. Not so much that the skin becomes red and irritated but more than simply getting it wet with the wipe. Remember the top layer of skin is made up of loosely connected layers of dead skin cells. Bacteria grow between the cells and you want to sterilize the site well enough to kill off as much of the bacteria as possible.

Scrub the entire area surrounding your intended site of insertion. This will remove the film of oil and loose dead skin allowing the transparent dressing to stick better.

LOCAL ANESTHESIA

If you are going to use local anesthesia do it at this point.

There are many different methods of inducing local analgesia for venipuncture. Unfortunately none are particularly widespread. Check your facilities policy. Some organizations require a physician's order for this, others do not.

This can be helpful with an extremely apprehensive patient that will not cooperate with the procedure.

Intradermally Injected Lidocaine

The quickest and most common method is to inject 1-2% solution of lidocaine subcutaneously for near instantaneous numbing. Commonly referred to as 'Novocain', this is the same anaesthetic that dentists use to numb the gums prior to a dental procedure.

Use a Tuberculin syringe to inject a small wheal of Lidocaine at the site where you intend to puncture the skin or just to the side of it. Although the patient will feel a slight prick from the initial injection of lidocaine, it should diminish their sensation of the larger—and more painful—puncture by the IV catheter. The Tuberculin syringe is 27G whereas the IV catheter is 18-22G.

Topical Anesthetics

Another method that does not require a separate injection involves applying a topical anesthetic. This includes EMLA (a mix of lidocaine and prilocaine), LMX (encapsulated lidocaine) and tetracaine. These creams or gels must be applied to the skin, wrapped in a non-occlusive dressing and left on for 30 minutes to one hour to become fully effective.

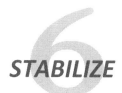

STABILIZE

Surface veins are not well anchored and prone to rolling. You will need to apply *counter-traction* when inserting the IV to prevent the vein from moving out of place. Do this by using your non-dominant hand to pull backwards on the skin surrounding the vein.

Deeper veins are held in place by the surrounding connective tissue. If the vein does not move at all when pushed side to side you may not need to apply much counter-traction.

If a vein rolls when you insert the IV, it's because you did not stabilize it sufficiently.

If you used your fingernail to make an impression on the patient's skin, be aware that the vein can roll underneath the skin. Thus it is important to stabilize the vein so it does not move from that position.

Stabilizing a Vein

Visualize where you will insert the needle and then use the thumb or fingers of your non-dominant hand to stretch the skin back. This method holds traction well but you may have difficulty inserting at a shallow angle since your fingers will get in the way.

1. **Adjust the patients arm to a position comfortable for you.**
2. **Place the index finger of your non-dominant hand an inch or two below the site**
3. **Applying counter-traction by using your index finger to pull the patient's skin back toward their hand.**
4. **Insert the IV over your finger into the vein**

If the vein is especially 'rolly' you may need to place your finger on the vein itself and pull back. This stabilizes the vein and prevents it from rolling when the needle is advanced. But be careful not to press too hard causing the vein to collapse.

Stabilizing a Shallow Vein

Shallow veins require a lower angle of insertion. You may notice that your thumb or fingers "get in the way" of the device forcing you to use a deeper angle. This method keeps your fingers out of the way but does not hold as traction as well.

1. Adjust the patients arm to a position comfortable for you.
2. Make a "C" with the thumb and index finger of your non-dominant hand.
3. Place your thumb and index finger on either side of the vein.
4. Use your thumb and index finger to pull back, stretching their skin toward their hand.
5. Your other three fingers should be out of the way above the site.
6. You will be able to insert the IV with as low an angle as necessary.

Stabilizing the Cephalic Vein (thumb side of forearm)

The cephalic vein is a large superficial vein that runs from the dorsal venous network of the hand, up along the lateral aspect of the forearm (thumb side) to the shoulder. It is usually easy to visualize and palpate although very likely to roll and must be stabilized well during venipuncture.

1. Adjust the patients arm to a position comfortable for you.
2. Have the patient make a fist and bend their wrist downward.
3. Grasp the patient's fist around the wrist and pull their skin toward their fingers.

Stabilizing Hand Veins

Veins in the hand are easily visualized and palpable. They are also excellent targets for a first or second attempt because even if a vein in the hand blows, the rest of the arm is still available for another attempt. To stabilize a vein in the hand:

1. Have the patient rest their elbow on the bed/stretcher with their arm standing up.
2. Have the patient bend their wrist so their palm faces downward.
3. Grasp the patient's fingers by placing your fingers underneath their fingers and your thumb just below their knuckles.
4. The patients fingers should be in-between your thumb and your fingers.
5. Use your thumb to pull down, stretching the patients skin over their knuckles

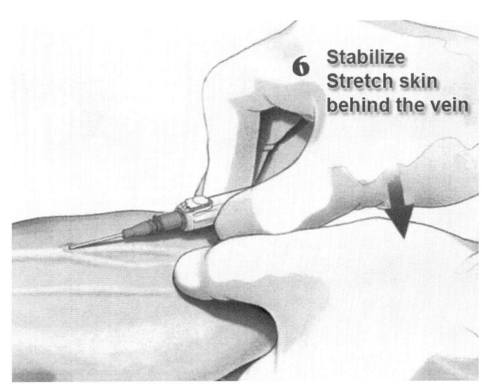

Figure 18 - Step 6: Stabilize and Stretch

7 INSERT THE NEEDLE

1. With your dominate hand hold the needle at the hub or grip pads.
2. Ensure that the bevel side is facing up.
3. Tell the patient that you will now insert the catheter.
4. With a smooth motion push the needle through the skin and into the vein until you see a flash of blood in the flashback chamber.
5. Pause and proceed to the next step.

When inserting the IV you will need to choose an appropriate angle and approach.

- The angle you insert will depend on the depth of the vein.
- The standard approach is through the top of the vein, but you can also enter through the side or directly into a bifurcation.

Pop!

While inserting the IV you will feel resistance at two points. The larger the needle, the more resistance you will feel. The first will occur as you press the needle through the patient's skin. You may encounter a lot of resistance in some male patients with very thick skin. You will need to aggressively push the needle through the skin.

Once the needle has passed through the skin it will enter the subcutaneous tissue. You will feel little to no resistance as you pass through this layer.

You will again feel a very subtle pop or moment of resistance as you pierce through the wall of the vein. At this point you should notice blood in the tubing or flashback chamber. The "pop" will be more obvious in large, healthy and/or thick veins. It may be less obvious or even absent in small, delicate fragile veins with thin walls.

Approaching the Vein:

Top Approach

This is the standard method to enter the vein. Position the tip of the needle directly on top of the vein. Push the needle down through the skin into the vein. Be sure to stop once you have entered the vein or you risk piercing through the back wall of the vein.

Side Approach

With this approach you will position the needle to the side of the vein. Push the needle through the skin towards the vein. This method reduces the risk of passing straight through a vein. You may also end up using this approach if you have inadvertently inserted the needle to the side of a vein or if the vein moves after you insert it from the top. You can still salvage the stick by switching to a side approach.

Through a Bifurcation

When presented with a bifurcation the standard approach is to insert the needle from the top just above the bifurcation. Alternatively, you can insert the needle directly into the bifurcation. Avoid this approach if a valve is located at the bifurcation.

Deciding on an Angle

The angle that you insert the IV will depend on the depth of the vein. Try to visualize the location of the vein and how the needle will enter it. Ideally, you want the IV to enter the vein as shallow as possible.

Most veins run parallel to the skin. With shallow superficial veins, you will want to insert the needle at a shallow angle and lower it even more when advancing. With deep veins, you need to insert at a deeper angle just to reach the vein; but since the vein runs parallel to the skin you must drop the angle after accessing the vein.

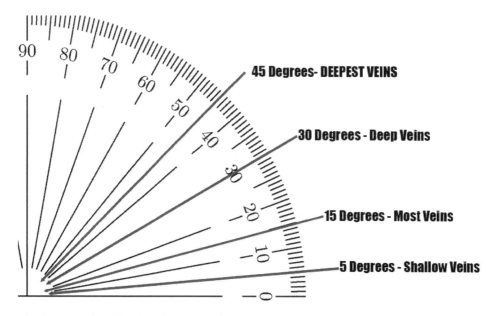

Shallow veins that bulge out from the skin require a very shallow angle, 15 degrees or less. The veins on the dorsal surface of the hand (back of the hand) as well as the cephalic vein (thumb side of forearm) often fall into this category.

Deep veins such as the AC (antecubital, at the bend of the elbow) will require a greater angle, 30 to 45 degrees.

The other veins of the forearm usually fall in between.

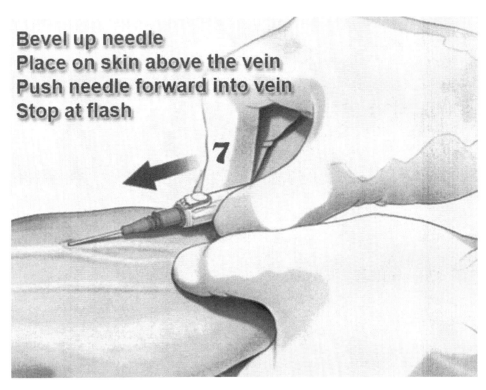

Figure 19 - Step 7: Push Needle Forward

8

WATCH FOR THE FLASH

LOWER YOUR ANGLE AND ADVANCE ANOTHER 1-2MM

RELEASE THE TOURNIQUET

1. **When you see the flash lower your angle so that the needle is nearly parallel to their arm or hand.**
2. **Then advance the needle another 1-2mm.**
3. **Now release the tourniquet with your non-dominate hand.**

The flash indicates that the **NEEDLE** is inside the vein **NOT** the **CATHETER**. This is why it is important to advance the needle another 1-2mm after visualizing the flash.

If you do not lower the angle you may pass through the back of the vein when advancing it.

Many IV rookies will see the flash, get excited and immediately attempt to advance the catheter.

Notice in the following graphic that the needle is inside the vein but the catheter is not. Also note that if you do not lower your angle to parallel with the vein you will push the needle right through the other side of the vein and it will blow. You may also notice that the bevel is facing to the side, not up; you always want the bevel facing up.

Tip!

Larger catheters have more space between the tip of the needle and the tip of the catheter than smaller needles.

With an 18G catheter you will need to advance another 2mm, with a small 22G catheter you only need to advance another 1mm.

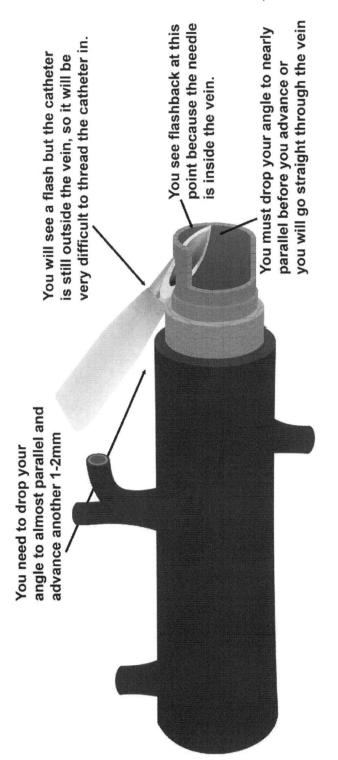

You will see a flash but the catheter is still outside the vein, so it will be very difficult to thread the catheter in.

You see flashback at this point because the needle is inside the vein.

You must drop your angle to nearly parallel before you advance or you will go straight through the vein

You need to drop your angle to almost parallel and advance another 1-2mm

Figure 20 - Lower Angle and Advance another 1-2mm

9 *THREAD THE CATHETER*

At this point *both* the tip of the needle *and* the tip of the catheter are inside the vein. You will now need to thread the rest of the catheter into the vein. The catheter is fully inside the vein when only the hub sticks out. There are several different methods to advancing the catheter:

The Two Handed Technique

1. You have already visualized flash, lowered your angle, advanced 1-2mm and released the tourniquet.
2. Continue holding the needle in place
3. With your non-dominant hand, grasp the hub of the catheter and slide it forward into the vein
4. Slowly withdraw the needle
5. Place your thumb on the hub of the catheter to hold it in place
6. Use your index finger to press down above the site to prevent blood from spilling out

The Single Handed Technique

1. You have already visualized flash, lowered your angle, advanced 1-2mm and released the tourniquet.
2. Continue holding the needle in place.
3. Use the index finger of the hand that is holding the needle to slide the catheter past the needle
4. Continue sliding the catheter until it is fully inside the vein.

With the above two techniques, be careful that you are only advancing the catheter into the vein and not the needle.

If the catheter is inside the vein it should be relatively easy and painless to advance it. Unlike the needle, the catheter is soft and flexible so it will be difficult to slide it in unless you are inside the vein.

- If the flashback was very small, you feel resistance and your patient is wincing in pain you may be threading the catheter in muscle or subcutaneous tissue.
- If the patient has very thick skin, you will feel more resistance while threading the catheter. You may have to advance the needle further and then thread the catheter.
- Resistance could also indicate that you are hitting against a valve or that the vein has collapsed. In this case you may still be able to salvage the IV by switching to the "floating technique."

The Straight Technique

With this method, you do not thread the catheter at all; you advance the entire needle into the vein. This technique is quicker but only works on straight superficial veins without valves. There is greater risk of piercing through the vein and blowing it since you are advancing the entire needle. This method can be helpful in a patient with thick skin where you would encounter significant resistance attempting to thread the catheter in.

1. You have already visualized flash and lowered your angle.
2. Instead of advancing just 1-2mm, advance the entire needle into the vein until only the hub of the catheter sticks out
3. Retract the needle while securing the hub and holding pressure above the site

The Float Technique

A basic overview is provided here, but we discuss this technique in greater detail in the next chapter.

This method involves threading, or 'floating', the catheter into the vein without the needle and while flushing. There is much less risk of puncturing through the vein with this technique. However it is critical to carefully secure the hub while removing the needle and attaching the flush/tubing. There is greater risk that the catheter will be pulled out before you are able to advance it, because at first only the tip of the catheter will be inside the vein.

1. You have already visualized flash, lowered your angle, advanced 1-2mm and released the tourniquet.
2. At this point you can either immediately retract the needle or attempt to thread the catheter until you meet resistance.
3. Retract the needle while securing the hub and holding pressure above the site
4. Connect tubing with a flush to the catheter.
5. Slowly flush while advancing the catheter.
6. Continue flushing and advancing until the catheter is inside the vein.

The following illustration depicts the single-handed technique. This works best with catheters that include a "push-tab".

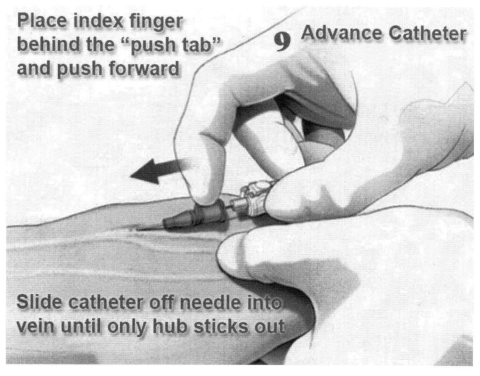

Place index finger behind the "push tab" and push forward

9 Advance Catheter

Slide catheter off needle into vein until only hub sticks out

Figure 21 - Step 9: Advance Catheter (using single-handed technique)

10 RETRACT THE NEEDLE

When the catheter is fully threaded in the vein you need to retract the needle without dislodging the catheter or allowing blood to spill out.

1. **The catheter is fully threaded in the vein.**
2. **(10A) Visualize where the tip of the catheter is and use your index or middle finger to press down at that spot.**
3. **(10B) Use the thumb or index finger of your other hand to secure the hub.**
4. **(10C) Slide the needle out or press the activator button to retract it.**

If you don't hold pressure above the site, blood will immediately flow out of the catheter and spill onto the patient. If this happens don't panic! Just release the tourniquet and put pressure and inch or two above the insertion site (about where the tip would be) to stop blood flow. You will then have to clean off the blood with an alcohol wipe before placing the dressing.

If you forgot to pull the tourniquet, the vein will still be pressurized and blood will rapidly pour out. Quickly pull the tourniquet and put pressure above the site.

If you pull the needle out, don't hold pressure and no blood flows out, there is a good chance that the stick was unsuccessful. You should attempt to aspirate and flush anyway to confirm since the IV may still be good.

The following three illustrations depict these steps in order. With experience you will learn to do all three steps simultaneously.

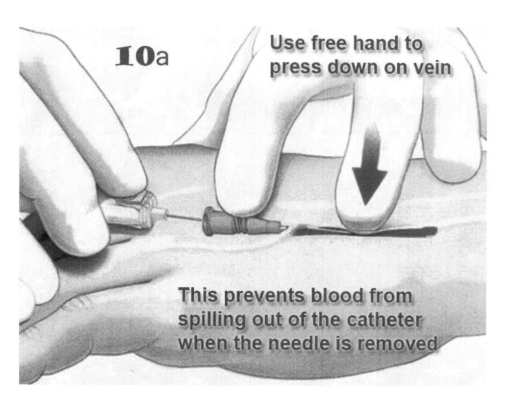

Figure 22 - Step 10a: Press Down on Vein

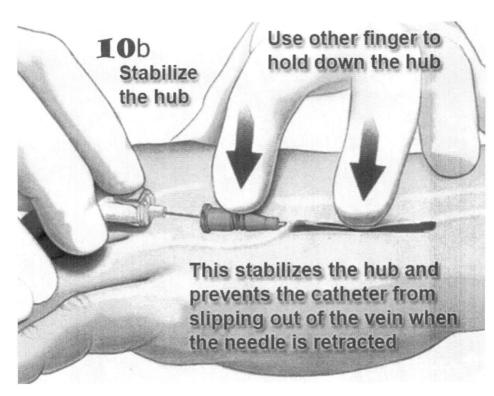

Figure 23 - Step 10b: Stabilize Hub

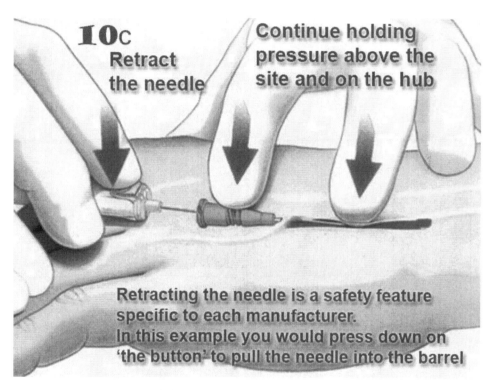

Figure 24 - Step 10c: Withdraw Needle

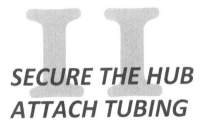

SECURE THE HUB
ATTACH TUBING

Use a small piece of tape to secure the hub and prevent the catheter from sliding out. You will only have one free hand, so this is why it is important to prepare the tape before you start.

Continue to hold pressure above the site until the tubing is attached.

If you haven't already released the tourniquet do so now or you risk blowing the vein when you flush.

VERIFY THE STICK IS GOOD

Aspirate the syringe just enough to see a flash of blood in the tubing and then flush the site with 10mL saline.

If the catheter is correctly placed you should see blood in the tubing when withdrawing and be able to flush without much resistance.

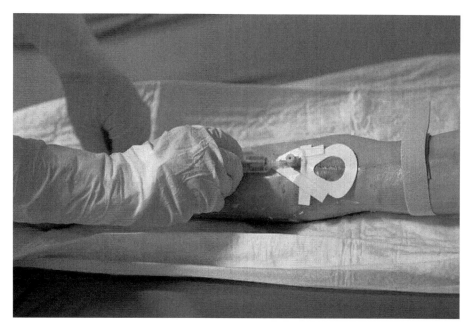

Figure 25 - Blood Aspirated

Any signs of a blown vein?

1. A bruise forming around the site of insertion.
2. Unable to aspirate blood
3. Meeting resistance when flushing
4. Swelling around site while flushing
5. Tissue is cool, tight, swollen around site after flushing.

A bruise forming or swelling while flushing are surefire signs of a blown vein. If you cannot aspirate and/or meet resistance while flushing, the vein may be blown or the catheter could just be pressed against a valve or the wall of the vein. Try to move the catheter a little while attempting to flush, and then try to aspirate again.

If the vein is blown, remove the catheter and at the same time press down on the puncture site with a piece of gauze and hold pressure for a few minutes to prevent a hematoma from forming. Don't forget to pull the tourniquet or the hematoma will rapidly enlarge.

See the chapter: *Veins that Blow* for more details.

13

SECURE THE SITE

Now that you verified the stick is good, secure the site with a transparent dressing (e.g. OpSite, Tegaderm, etc.).

Sign and date the dressing to ensure that it will be changed within 96hrs.

Thank the patient, clean up and don't forget to document the insertion.

Tip!

Always double check that you removed the tourniquet prior to leaving the room.

Make this a habit.

"THE FLOATING TECHNIQUE"

The standard technique is appropriate for routine uncomplicated IV insertions. Certain situations call for an alternative approach, the "floating technique" is one of these. This technique is useful when attempting to access valvular, torturous or collapsed veins—that is veins with many valves, veins that twist and turn or flat veins. It is also helpful when you have accessed a vein, obtained flash but are unable to advance because of too much resistance.

This technique is good for inexperienced users who tend to blow veins because you are much less likely to puncture straight through the vein to the opposite side.

Floating the catheter involves inserting the needle just enough to get at least the tip of the catheter inside the vein. The needle is then withdrawn with the remainder of the catheter still exposed. A flush is attached to the hub of the catheter; and the catheter is advanced forward while slowly flushing.

Why Float?

The standard technique assumes that you have located and avoided any valves and that the vein is already sufficiently distended to allow the catheter to advance freely. Flushing while advancing the catheter causes any valves in the way to open as well as causing the vein to fill and expand. This creates more room for the catheter to advance.

Patients who are dehydrated or otherwise hypovolemic may not have sufficiently distended veins. If the vein is empty/collapsed it will be difficult to tread the catheter in. By flushing, the vein fills up causing it to expand. This creates enough room for the catheter to advance forward. Attempting to advance a catheter on a collapsed/flat vein is nearly impossible because there is no space within the lumen of the vein. The catheter ends up just scraping against the wall of the vein causing it to bend. If you attempt to advance with the needle still in place the needle will puncture through the vein causing it to blow. Flushing expands the vein and opens any valves in the way allowing the catheter to advance with much less resistance.

Step by Step

The float technique uses the same basic steps as the standard technique. Prepare your equipment, apply tourniquet, scrub the site, stabilize the vein by holding traction to the skin with your non-dominate hand while holding the needle with your dominate hand.

1. Insert the needle.
2. Watch for flash.
3. Lower your angle and advance another 1-2mm.
4. If you can, attempt to thread the catheter until you meet resistance.
5. Release the tourniquet.
6. Secure the hub with the thumb or index finger of your other hand.
7. Put pressure above the site with your index or middle finger. *sometimes you may not have enough hands to do this, in that case just clean any blood that spills
8. Retract the needle while securing the hub and holding pressure above the site.
9. Connect tubing with a flush to the catheter.
10. Release holding pressure above the site but keep the hub secure.
11. Slowly flush while advancing the catheter.
12. Continue flushing and advancing until the catheter is fully inside the vein.
13. Secure the site and apply a dressing.

Insertion of the needle is the same: use an appropriate angle of insertion, watch for a flash, then lower the angle to almost parallel with the skin and advance the needle another 1-2mm to push the tip of the catheter inside the vein. These steps are the same as with the standard technique.

The difference occurs when advancing the catheter. With the standard technique, you would thread the catheter past the needle fully into the vein until only the hub is sticking out and then retract the needle.

To float the catheter in you only partially advance it and then STOP. You want to try to thread it a little because the catheter can easily slip out before you have a chance to float it in since only 1-2mm of it is inside the vein at first. However if you meet resistance you can stop and attempt to float it the rest of the way.

Remember to only advance the catheter and not the needle! Part of the catheter will remain outside the vein and resting on the patients (hopefully well sterilized) skin.

Tip!

Remember the difference between advancing the needle and advancing/threading the catheter.

When you advance the needle you push the entire device forward.

To advance just the catheter you push it past the needle into the vein, the needle should remain stationary and not move forward.

At this point release the tourniquet and prepare to withdraw the needle. Prior to withdrawing the needle you will need to use your index (or middle) finger to place pressure above the site to prevent blood from spilling out of the catheter. Use your thumb (or index finger) of the same hand to stabilize the hub of the catheter.

With your index finger holding pressure above the site and your thumb securing the hub, use your other hand to withdraw and remove the needle. Set it aside and grab the tubing with flush and secure it to the hub of the catheter. When the tubing/flush is secured to the hub you can release pressure above the site but continue to hold the catheter securely.

It is critical that you keep the hub of the catheter secure during this procedure. Depending on how far you were able to initially thread it, only part of the catheter will be inside the vein. If you were unable to tread it at all then only 1-2mm will be inside the vein. The slightest movement can dislodge the catheter from the vein causing it to blow. Sometimes you may have to forgo holding pressure and focus on just securing the hub while retracting the needle and immediately attaching the tubing. In this case some blood may spill out of the catheter in between steps. Ignore it for the moment, attach the tubing/flush and float the catheter in. You can clean up the blood afterwards.

You can do without the tubing and attach a 10cc flush with a needleless valve/hub directly to the hub of the catheter but using extension tubing provides more flexibility and decreases the likelihood of the catheter being pulled out of the vein accidentally.

At this point you should have the catheter attached to the tubing with flush but part of the catheter still exposed outside the vein.

Remember that since the catheter is not fully inside the vein it is very important to hold it securely because the slightest movement could cause it to pull out of the vein.

Now slowly flush the catheter with one hand while advancing it with the other. Carefully watch for any signs of infiltration such as swelling of the tissue around the site. Continue to flush while advancing the catheter until it is fully inside the vein and only the hub extends outside. Aspirate the flush and observe for blood return to confirm that you are indeed within the vein. Attach a second flush and flush the catheter again while observing for swelling or other signs of infiltration. Then apply tape and dressing as with any other IV.

Prevent Contamination

One concern with the floating technique is the potential for infection because part of the catheter remains exposed to the patient's skin. To mitigate this risk it is important to thoroughly scrub the skin with alcohol, or ideally a CHG wipe, prior to insertion ALL THE TIME. It is also important never to touch the catheter itself since that is the portion that will be inside the patient's body.

VEINS THAT BLOW

What does it mean to "Blow a Vein"?

In a successful IV stick the wall of the vein should remain intact with only a single puncture through which the catheter enters. A blown vein indicates that the venous wall has ruptured and blood is spilling out into the surrounding tissue.

Too much pressure

If the walls of the vein are weak they may rupture the moment the needle punctures through.

The vein ruptures when the catheter punctures the wall because of too much pressure exerted against the walls of the vein. The culprit in this case is a tourniquet that is too tight on veins that are too fragile. You need to adjust the tightness or do without it completely. Healthy veins need a tight tourniquet to fully dilate; however, fragile veins will fully dilate with a much looser tourniquet. Try loosening the tourniquet until you notice the vein is losing distension. Then tighten it just enough to be sufficiently distended but not anymore.

Skewering the Vein

This is probably the most common reason a vein blows during insertion.

The needle may have entered the vein properly but then advanced too far, passing straight through to the other side, essentially skewering it. This is more common with smaller veins. You need to advance enough that both the needle and the tip of the catheter are inside the lumen of the vein but not so far that it passes through and out the other side. Smaller veins have less room for error.

Entering at too steep of an angle will also increase the probability of passing straight through the vein.

You can identify this by the characteristic small flash that then stops partially up the catheter—a "half flash!" The flash started when you entered the vein but then stopped when the needle passed through the other side of the vein. If you withdraw the needle a little the flash will return—and you may get a good blood return and be able to flush—but the vein is blown because of the hole that you created on the other side.

To overcome this you will need to slow down your approach.

This also happens when if you forget to lower your angle before continuing to advance.

Remember to lower your angle after the flashback. You want to advance the needle parallel to the vein.

See the following graphic: Figure 26 on the next page for a visualization of this.

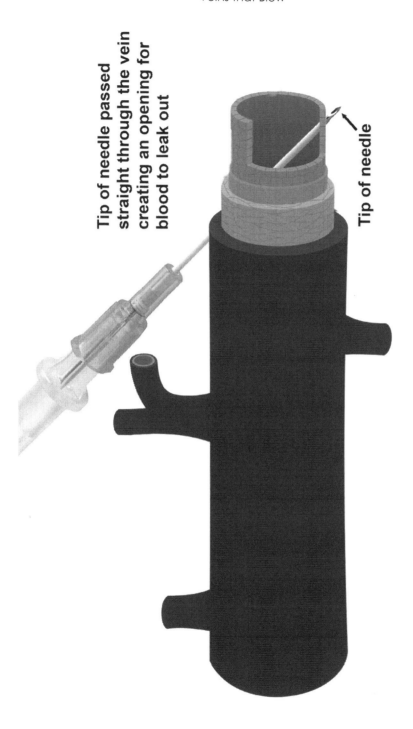

Tip of needle passed straight through the vein creating an opening for blood to leak out

Tip of needle

Figure 26 - Skewering the Vein

In and out

In this case the needle entered the vein properly but then got pulled out. Blood will start flowing out of the puncture blowing the vein. Similar to skewering the vein you may see a small "half flash".

There is nothing that you can do to salvage this. If you attempt to reenter the vein you will create a second opening.

Not far enough

This happens when you attempt to thread the catheter before it is in the vein.

Remember that the needle extends 1-2mm past the catheter and both the needle and the tip of the catheter need to be inside the vein before you start to thread the catheter in. If you stop advancing the needle the moment you get a flash it will be difficult to thread the catheter in. Unlike the needle, the catheter is flexible and bends easily. It is also wider than the needle (since it surrounds the needle).

This is a common problem with IV rookies: they see the flash, get excited and immediately retract the needle and attempt to thread the catheter in. Or you see the flash and fear passing straight through the vein so you don't advance far enough. To overcome this you just need to remember to lower your angle, advance 1-2mm *after* the flash and *then* thread the catheter in.

The following graphic: Figure 27 depicts this problem.

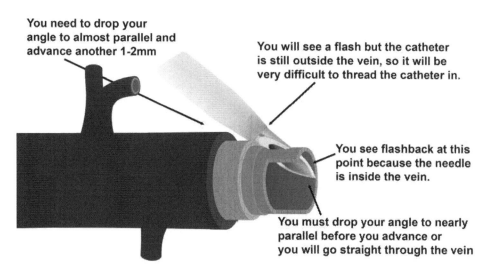

You need to drop your angle to almost parallel and advance another 1-2mm

You will see a flash but the catheter is still outside the vein, so it will be very difficult to thread the catheter in.

You see flashback at this point because the needle is inside the vein.

You must drop your angle to nearly parallel before you advance or you will go straight through the vein

Figure 27 - Needle in Vein

Know when the vein is blown

When inserting an IV, it is important to be able to identify if the vein blows. There is no point to salvage a blown vein but it is not always apparent. The site where the vein ruptured should immediately swell. If the vein was superficial you may notice a bruise forming. However the discoloration does not always immediately follow the swelling.

You can test the IV by flushing it. If the vein did blow you should feel resistance and the site should swell if you flush. Assess the skin for signs of infiltration. Cool and tight skin around the site is one indication. The flush is room temperature so should feel much cooler than the patient's body temperature. The small infiltration will also cause the skin to feel tighter than surrounding tissue.

VALVES

Gravity naturally pulls blood towards the ground. Arteries overcome this by the pumping action of the heart and the muscular artery itself. The blood in veins is pumped passively by skeletal muscle movement and breathing but under very little pressure. Veins within the limbs contain the most valves and they work to prevent blood from flowing backwards. Unfortunately they also interfere with IV sticks.

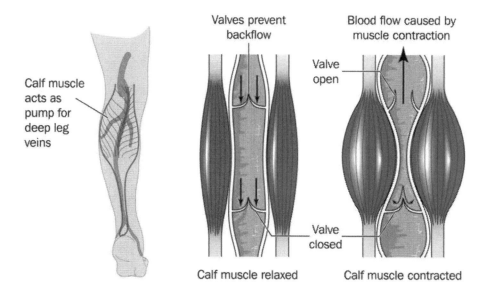

Figure 28 - Illustration of how blood is pumped in veins

When a tourniquet is tightened around the patient, venous blood flow past the tourniquet is largely occluded. Blood continues to flow into the limb through the artery (unless the tourniquet is so tight that arterial blood flow is impeded as well). This blood makes its way to the tissues and then into the veins. Blood is mostly unable to flow out past the tourniquet but also cannot flow backwards because the valves close. As the veins swell with blood, they become distended making them easy to see and feel.

An IV inserted behind one of these valves will be difficult to advance since the catheter tip will bend when pressed against the closed valve. It will also occlude the tip of the catheter and prevent blood from being withdrawn. If the needle itself punctures the valve, the vein may blow.

Thus it is important to identify valves when selecting an IV site.

They are often found at junctions were two veins join together into one. Valves also appear as raised bumps along the length of the vein. If you carefully palpate the vein you should be able to feel the subtle difference between the smooth length of the vein and the bump of the valve. The valve will have a slightly denser/harder consistency than the rest of the vein. It will also not collapse as easily and will not feel as bouncy when compressed.

Tip!

When the tourniquet is tightened around the patient's arm, all the valves close.

The Float Technique pushes the valves open and allows the catheter to slide past a valve.

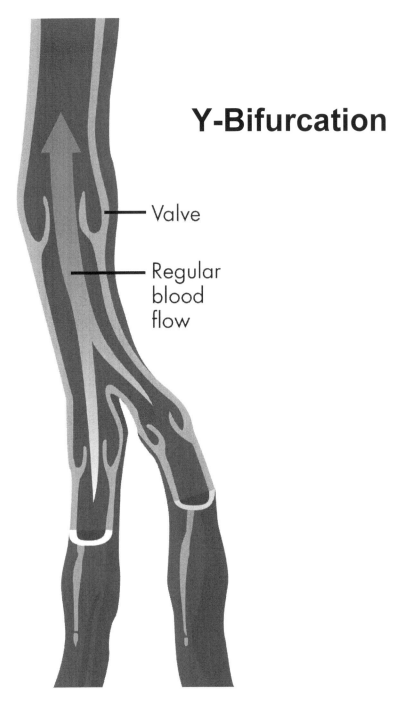

Y-Bifurcation

Valve

Regular
blood
flow

Figure 29 – Y-Bifurcation of Normal Vein and Valves

To confirm presence of a valve try the following method:

1. Place tourniquet causing veins to distend (swell up)
2. Identify a vein you want to evaluate
3. Use your thumb to place pressure on the vein
4. Place your index finger next to your thumb
5. Spread your index finger out proximal (upward, toward the shoulder) along the length of the vein while pressing down
6. This opens the valves ahead and pushes all the blood out of that segment of the vein causing it to flatten.
7. Release your index finger but continue holding pressure with your thumb.
8. When you release your index finger, a section of the vein just above your thumb should remain flat. But blood should flow backward and fill up the rest of the vein up to the nearest valve
9. That point where it goes from flat to distended marks the location of the valve
10. When you release your thumb you should notice the flat section immediately fill up
11. You will be clear of any valves as long as the IV catheter is shorter than the flat section and you insert it just above where you held pressure with your thumb

VENIPUNCTURE IN ELDERLY PATIENTS

Venipuncture in older adults present some unique challenges. Although their veins are often more visible due to loss of surrounding tissue, they are also thinner, more fragile and prone to rupture and infiltration.

- Loss of collagen with age causes the skin to lose elasticity and makes it thin, fragile and susceptible to tears and bruising.
- Loss of the subcutaneous tissue that anchors veins in place makes them more prone to rolling aside when the needle is inserted.
- The walls of the veins themselves become weaker, more fragile and prone to rupturing when pierced by the needle.
- The elderly have a weakened immune system and are more susceptible to infection. Strict aseptic technique is a must.
- Large hematomas can quickly develop because of longer bleeding times, either naturally or due to concurrent treatment with blood thinners. These patients require pressure to be held for longer when a vein blows.
- Elderly patients are at higher risk of fluid volume overload from IV fluid therapy. Monitor the patient closely for crackles in the lower lobes, rapid respirations and shortness of breath.

Loosen the tourniquet

Tightening a tourniquet around thin fragile skin can cause it to tear. It can also cause petechiae or the formation of a hematoma.

A tight tourniquet will build up more pressure in the vein than necessary. This will cause the vein to immediately blow when pierced by the needle.

The tourniquet only needs to be tight enough to cause the veins to distend so that you can palpate them and insert the catheter. In the elderly, you can achieve the same result with a much looser tourniquet.

Any vein will blow if you puncture straight through it to the other side but if you notice that the vein seems to blow the moment you access it and get flashback try loosening the tourniquet just enough to keep the veins distended but no more.

Don't use the tourniquet

Many elderly patients have veins that are sufficiently distended even without a tourniquet. If you can visualize *and* palpate the vein without the tourniquet on then you probably do not need to apply one. The vein is less likely to blow without the tourniquet.

Use a BP cuff

If a tourniquet is necessary to properly distend the veins try using a blood pressure cuff instead. The BP cuff allows for better control of pressure and spreads that pressure out over a larger surface area. Inflate the cuff to 40 to 60 mmHg.

Stabilize the vein with traction

Superficial veins in the elderly are especially prone to rolling because of the erosion of connective and subcutaneous tissue that once held it in place. Apply counter traction to the skin surrounding the vein or even the vein itself to prevent it from moving out of the way.

Lower your angle of insertion

Elderly veins are closer to the surface of the skin because of thinning of the subcutaneous tissue. The insertion angle must be very shallow to ensure that the needle does not puncture through to the posterior side of the vein. When inserting the needle, it should be almost parallel to the surface of the skin.

Use a smaller catheter

A smaller catheter may be more appropriate for elderly patients. Their veins are smaller and unable to accommodate large catheters. Try using a 22G or 24G unless a larger one is specifically warranted.

INFILTRATION AND EXTRAVASATION

Infiltration of any fluid or medication is bad, but some are REALLY BAD. This is the difference between infiltration and extravasation.

Infiltration

Infiltration is the leakage of any medication or fluid outside the vein and into the surrounding tissue. This generally results in swelling, pallor, coolness of the skin and discomfort/pain in the area.

Mild to moderate infiltration will generally clear up on its own without permanent injury. The swelling will slowly diminish over time as the infiltrate is absorbed by the body. Severe infiltration can cause compartment syndrome and must be dealt with emergently. This occurs when so much fluid infiltrates that the nerves and arteries become compressed.

Extravasation

Extravasation is the infiltration of a fluid or medication that is so irritating to the surrounding tissue that it causes blisters to form or even necrosis.

These fluids and medications are called **vesicants**. Severe extravasation can lead to the need for debridement and grafting or even amputation.

The mechanism of damage as well as treatment is specific to each vesicant. Highly acidic (vancomycin) or alkaline medications chemically damage the surrounding tissue and cytotoxic medications (such as chemotherapy) directly kill living cells. Whereas vasopressors (such as Levophed® and dopamine) cause severe vasoconstriction cutting off blood supply to the tissue.

You need to know if the medication you are giving has the potential to cause serious extravasation injury and pay more careful attention to them. Ideally vesicants should be administered through a central line such as a PICC. If infusing through a peripheral IV, the site must be monitored frequently for any signs of infiltration.

Tip!

Know if the medication or fluid you are infusing is a vesicant.

These infusions must be monitored more carefully to prevent extravasation injury.

Flush these lines frequently to assess patency.

Managing simple infiltration

It is important to distinguish infiltration from extravasation. If you are certain that the fluid or medication is not a vesicant you can treat it as a simple infiltration.

1. **Stop the infusion**
2. **Disconnect the tubing**
3. **Aspirate the site to remove as much residual medication as possible**
4. **Remove the IV**
5. **Elevate the site for 24 to 48 hours**
6. **Place a warm compress on the site**
7. **Continue to monitor the site and assess pulses and sensation**

Elevating the site helps to drain the infiltrate by increasing absorption into the capillaries.

A warm compress causes vasodilation which helps dilute the infiltrate, spreading it over a larger area as well as absorbing it.

Stop the infusion! But don't pull the catheter (yet)

It is important to know what to do if you suspect extravasation. You will want to refer to your facility's policy and procedures as well as informing the physician. Treatment will be specific to the medication as well as the extent of the extravasation.

In general, you will want to immediately stop the infusion and disconnect the tubing. Even though the IV has infiltrated, DO NOT remove it just yet, you may need to infuse an antidote to neutralize the vesicant or normal saline to dilute it.

If you suspect extravasation:

1. **Immediately stop the infusion**
2. **Disconnect the tubing**
3. **Aspirate the site to remove as much residual medication as possible***
4. **Do NOT remove the IV**
5. **Do NOT flush the site**
6. **Mark and measure the extravasated area**
7. **Notify the attending physician**
8. **Administer an antidote, as ordered**
9. **Apply hot or cold pack****

*Often times you will not be able to aspirate anything

**A hot pack will cause vasodilation helping to dilute the vesicant by spreading it. A cold pack will cause vasoconstriction preventing the vesicant from spreading. You will want to place a cold pack on tissue extravasated by DNA-binding cytotoxic vesicants (these are specific chemotherapy agents). All others will benefit from a hot pack.

Common vesicant medications

The following lists common vesicant medications, but is by no means all inclusive:

- Most chemotherapy agents
- Potassium Chloride
- Dopamine
- Norepinephrine (Levophed®)
- Dobutamine
- Vasopressin
- Phenytoin (Dilantin®)
- Propofol
- TPN (Total Parenteral Nutrition)
- Contrast Agents (in Radiology)
- Diazepam (Valium®)
- Vancomycin
- Promethazine (Phenergan®)

TIPS AND TRICKS

Don't let the patient feel that you are not confident.

Walk into the room and look confident, even if you are new and have yet to successfully start an IV. No patient wants to hear, "This is my first time" or worse, "I haven't had much luck lately." If you miss or blow the vein, the patient will still feel more comfortable knowing that you are competent. Even if you missed or blew the last 6 attempts, let them think that you are confident. You are not performing surgery or some life threatening procedure. You are not going to cause permanent harm from missing or blowing a vein, it may be a little uncomfortable and they may end up with a bruise but this is how skills are passed down from one generation to the next.

If you are not confident ask a more experienced colleague to come with you to provide support and coaching.

Don't be afraid to ask for help. IV catheterization is one of the more difficult skills that a RN, LVN or EMT will have to learn. Most people will miss or blow several attempts in a row and it takes months to years to improve and truly become an expert. If you are just starting out it can be very helpful to have someone else with you to guide you through it and let you know if you are missing a step or doing something wrong. It can also be helpful because they can reassure (and distract) the patient while you focus on the IV.

Use a penlight to assess for infiltration.

Shine a penlight onto the swollen area and look for a diffuse halo of light to confirm infiltration. Then shine the penlight in the same area on the other arm. Compare the two: if the vein infiltrated with clear fluids running the halo will be larger because light is able to pass more easily through the infiltrated tissue.

Use an alcohol wipe to help search for good veins.

The alcohol wipe is not just for sterilizing the site prior to insertion, it can also be helpful while searching for good veins. After you place the tourniquet use an alcohol wipe to rub potential sites. Not only will the rubbing action induce the vein to distend but the alcohol itself will cause the skin to glisten making the vein more visible.

If the vein is small, you can leave the tourniquet tied while threading the catheter.

Small veins may collapse when the tourniquet is removed. This could result in resistance while threading the catheter. Sometimes it is helpful to leave the tourniquet in place as you thread the catheter. The tourniquet will keep the vein distended providing more room for the catheter to advance. If you have already released the tourniquet and are then having difficulty threading, reapply it to the patient, or switch to the floating technique.

If you touch the vein after cleaning it, you need to clean it again.

Everyone does it. They will find a good vein, have everything ready with needle in hand and just before puncture, touch the vein one last time. Don't do this! The whole point of scrubbing the skin with alcohol or CHG wipe is to sterilize it; you break that sterility when you touch the site again. If you cannot resist the urge and end up touching the vein, you will need to wipe it again. Try marking the site by pressing your fingernail into the skin directly over the vein were you want to insert the IV. This will leave an impression that you can use to guide placing the needle.

Don't forget to apply traction behind the vein.

Often times IVs are missed because traction was not applied behind the vein. Without traction superficial veins will roll away when hit by the needle. It can sometimes be difficult to apply traction because you are trying to insert at a shallow angle and your hand or fingers get in the way. Try different positions or using your thumb and index finger to make a "C," with the IV device in between. This is especially important with "rolly" veins.

Deeper veins are stronger and more stable than superficial veins.

Shallow veins are more likely to roll because they are not anchored down as well by the connective tissue that surrounds it. They are also thinner and thus more likely to blow or infiltrate. Deep veins are often difficult to visualize so you must rely on palpation to discover them. They will feel "bouncy" or "spongy" and should spring back when pressed compared to the surrounding tissue. This is something that you really have to practice to get a good feel for.

Never leave the patient after placing the tourniquet.

Only place the tourniquet when you are ready to search for the vein and take it off after inserting the needle or when you notice the vein is blown. Never leave the patient to fetch supplies with the tourniquet left on. It is always safer to remove it and place it again. If you notice that the vein is blown, withdraw the needle and immediately remove the tourniquet and place pressure around the puncture site. This will prevent an unnecessarily large bruise from forming.

Use a smaller catheter in a large vein for irritating infusions.

Infusions such as Amiodarone, Potassium, Phenytoin, Dextrose and other vesicants irritate the vein, sometimes leading to phlebitis. In these patients it can be helpful to place a small catheter (22G) in a larger vein (such as the AC). Larger veins have greater blood flow to diffuse the fluids and carry them away from the site.

Wear a set of gloves one size smaller than you normally do.

The tighter fit of the gloves will enable you to better feel the subtle characteristics of the vein. Some older—scratch that—more experienced nurses/EMTs were taught to tear off the tip of the glove covering the index finger to help with feeling the vein while inserting the IV. This is not recommended and is a breach of standard precautions. It exposes the patient to risk of contamination from your finger as well as exposing you to risk of infection from their blood. It is perfectly acceptable—and even encouraged—to feel the patient's skin and veins prior to insertion without gloves on, but always don gloves prior to the actual insertion.

There are two painful moments during venipuncture.

When inserting an IV, there are really only two points where it should be painful: the moment the needle punctures through the upper layer of skin and then again when the needle punctures through the wall of the vein. After puncturing the skin, the patient should not feel as much pain while the needle passes through the subcutaneus tissue. This gives you some time to "explore" for the vein if you do not hit it immediately. The patient should also not feel much pain while the catheter is being advanced into the vein.

Decrease your angle.

Only deep veins that you cannot visualize require a steep angle and NO vein will need an angle greater than 45 degrees. If you see a "half flash"—that is a small flash that then stops, you are probably passing straight through the vein. Most veins run parallel to the skin so your angle should be less than 30 degrees. Look back at the chapter: *Veins that Blow* for illustrations of this.

And always remember to drop your angle to nearly parallel (0 degrees) when you obtain flashback.

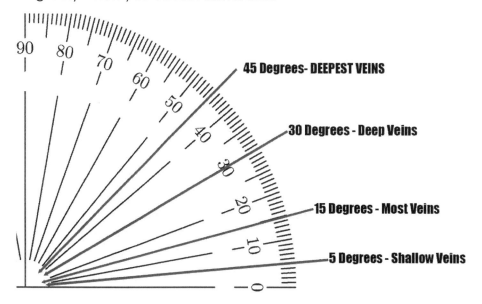

45 Degrees- DEEPEST VEINS

30 Degrees - Deep Veins

15 Degrees - Most Veins

5 Degrees - Shallow Veins

There should be minimal resistance when advancing the catheter inside the vein.

One of my classmates started an IV on me the first time and missed the vein but attempted to advance the catheter anyway. There was a lot of resistance and she could only push it about 2-4mm. Our professor was watching and asked me what it felt like, I said it felt like something was tearing or ripping… she told us that was because she was advancing the catheter inside or just above my muscle tissue!

Sometimes you will meet resistance while threading the catheter in the vein. It could be that you are hitting a valve or the vein is small and not sufficiently distended. If you are sure that you are in fact inside the vein, switch to the "float technique."

Don't blame your patient—or yourself for missing or blowing a vein.

Don't blame your patient by telling them you missed because their vein rolled out of the way or that it blew because they are on Coumadin®. Just say that you did not get it this time and you are going to start one more time. If you don't get it on your second attempt tell them you will call in an expert. Equally important is not to blame yourself. You will miss and blow a lot of veins when you are first starting out. Everyone learns through practice that is just how it is. And even experts will miss and blow easy veins every now and then.

END

Well that's all folks! If you made it this far you are that much closer to becoming an IV pro. But you will never become an expert at anything from just reading a book. You need to practice what you learn. Go out there; walk up to your patient with the confidence that you got this! Don't let failure discourage you. If you blow 10 veins in a row, don't give up; ask for help and keep trying.

Thank you for making it to the end. We hope you enjoyed this text and learned some valuable skills along the way.

If you have any questions or concerns please contact us at rapidresponsern@gmail.com. Please feel free to let us know of any typos, mistakes, omissions or anything that you think should be added to this text.

APPENDIX

Gauges

As you can see a 16G needle is twice as wide as a 22G.

SPECIFICATIONS				
Gauge	Colour Code	Ext. Dia. mm	Length mm	Flow Rate ml/min
14G	Orange	2.1	45	240
16G	Grey	1.8	45	180
18G	Green	1.3	32/45	90
20G	Pink	1.1	32	60
22G	Blue	0.9	25	36
24G	Yellow	0.7	19	20
26G	Violet	0.6	19	13

Vesicant Medications and Antidote

Vesicant Medication	Antidote
Aminophylline Calcium solutions Contrast media Concentrated dextrose Etoposide Nafcillin Potassium solutions Teniposide TPN Vinblastine Vincristine Vindesine	**Hyaluronidase**—15 units/mL 0.2 mL subcutaneous injection near site of extravasation
Dactinomycin	**Ascorbic acid**—50mg
Daunorubicin	**Hydrocortisone sodium succinate**—100 mg/mL Inject 50 to 200 mg
Dobutamine Dopamine Epinephrine Metaraminol Norepinephrine	**Phentolamine**—5 to 10 mg Dilute in 10 to 15 mL normal saline Administer up to 12 hours after extravasation
Mechlorethamine	**Sodium thiosulfate** 10%—10 mL

Made in the USA
Middletown, DE
10 October 2023

40591981R00073